Yoga

For Fitness

Monique Joiner Siedlak

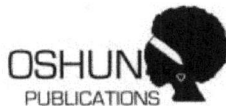

OSHUN
PUBLICATIONS

Printed in the United States of America

Second Edition 2018

ISBN-13: 978-1-948834-38-4

Publisher
www.oshunpublications.com

Disclaimer
All the material contained in this book is provided for educational and informational purposes only. No responsibility can be taken for any results or outcomes resulting from the use of this material. While every attempt has been made to provide information that is both accurate and effective, the author does not assume any responsibility for the accuracy or use/misuse of this information.

Notice

This book is not intended as a substitute for the medical advice of physicians. The reader should regularly consult a physician or therapist in matters relating to his/her health and particularly with respect to any symptoms that may require diagnosis or medical attention.

Yoga Poses Photos

Pixabay.com

Freepik.com

Dreamstime.com

Other Books in the Series

Table of Contents

Introduction to This Book

Working out is good for your body. It helps you get fit. However, who said yoga doesn't help in giving you a fit body? Yoga practitioners swear that yoga is a very effective and relaxing way to help your body get fit and healthy. Once you get the hang of yoga poses and get flexible, you can tackle the hardest of yoga poses for additional benefits.

For example; you can get flexible which can help prevent minor injuries, it can relieve you of certain pains like period pains, and it can even help your mind relax. A relaxed mind is key for you to be motivated enough to get fit. Your body literally reacts to the emotional state of your mind.

Yoga is better than going to a gym. You don't need to be lifting extra weights when you can do it all at your home with yoga. Yoga is also a better alternative to cardio. Yoga helps you appreciate your body and makes you realize how special it is. It motivates you to take better care of your body by eating healthy and staying positive.

Boat Pose (Navasana)

The Boat Pose is a great challenging yoga pose, but also a beneficial one. It builds core strength, stability, and awareness of posture, strengthening the abdominal and hip muscles.

How to Do

Start in a seated posture with your knees bent and your feet flat on the floor. Raise your feet off the floor. Maintain your knees bent at the beginning. Bring your shins parallel to the floor. This is the Half Boat Pose.

Your torso will want to instinctively fall back, but do not let your spine round.

If you can do so without losing the form of your upper body, straighten out your legs to a forty-five-degree angle. You want to hold your torso as vertical as possible so it creates a V shape with the legs.

Roll your shoulders backward and straighten your arms approximately parallel to the floor with your palms spun up. Balance on the sitting bones. Stay for at least five breaths.

Benefits

Builds strength and steadiness at the body's core and intensely challenges the abdomen, spine, and hip flexors.

Tip

You can, if it helps you to hold your spine straight, hold the backs of your thighs with your hands.

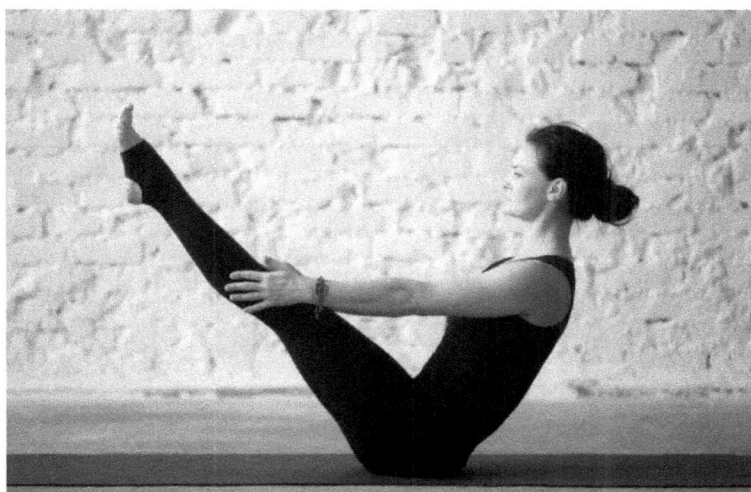

Dolphin Plank Pose (Makara Adho Mukha Svanasana)

The Dolphin Plank Pose is an intermediate level invigorating yoga pose that aids in toning the abdominal muscles.

How to Do

Begin in Downward Facing Dog. Move your weight forward so that your shoulders are over your wrists.

Lower your forearms, One by one, to the floor with your palms facing down. Place your elbows where your hands were, and spread your fingers wide. With your heels over your toes, you want your body to be in one straight line.

Draw your abdomen to your spine. Keeping the muscles in your glutes relaxed, draw your shoulders away from your ears, and stare between your hands.

Hold this for five whole breaths. At that time, come back onto your hands and press back into Downward Facing Dog.

Benefits

The Dolphin Plank Pose builds your strength in your shoulders arms and abdomen.

Tips

Rest your forehead on a block set between your forearms to relieve any neck tension you may have.

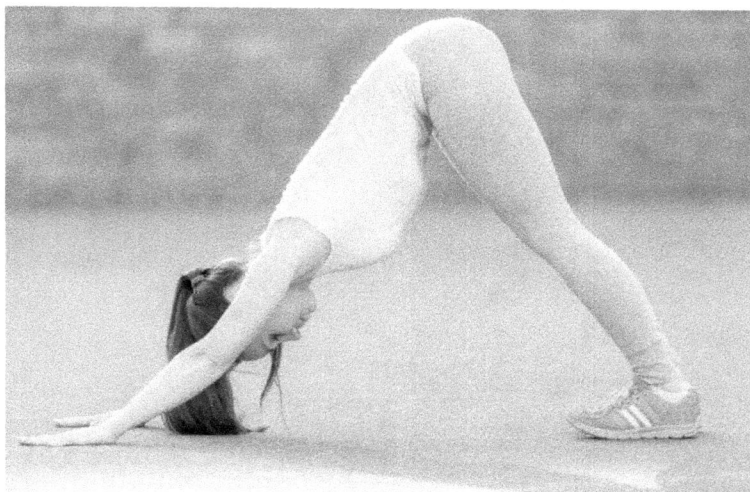

Extended Side Angle Pose (Utthita Parsvakonasana)

The Extended Side Angle Pose is a standing pose that stretches your legs, knees, hips, and ankles while increasing and improving endurance and stamina.

How to Do

Begin in the Mountain Pose. Turn to the right and lengthen your arms sideways to shoulder height with your palms facing down. Move your feet as wide apart as your wrists. Bring into line your heels.

Turn your left leg and foot outward ninety degrees so your toes point to the top of your mat. Bend your left knee until your left thigh is equal to the floor. Keeping your left knee directly over your heel, turn in your right toes to some extent. Line up the heel of your left foot with the arch of your right foot. Keeping your back leg straight, inhale and pull your right hip somewhat forward.

Do not turn your body in the direction of your left leg and keep your torso open to the right. Look out across the top of your left middle finger. This is the Warrior Two pose.

Exhale and lower your left arm so your forearm rests on your left thigh.

Extend your right arm up towards the ceiling, and then spread your arm over the top of your head. Your right bicep must be over your right ear, and your fingertips should be reaching in the same direction with your front toes pointing. Keep your chest, hips, and legs in one straight line, extended over your front leg.

Tilt your head to look up toward the ceiling. Keep your breathing smooth, your throat lax and your face relaxed.

To intensify the pose, lower your front hand to the floor, by placing your palm next to the inside arch of your front foot. Placing your front hand on the outside of your front foot will give you a greater chest and shoulder opening. You can also rest your front hand on a yoga block.

Make certain that your front knee does not drop inwardly. Keeping your front thigh on the outside turning with your knee, drawn it to some extent toward the baby toe of your front foot. Press firmly through the outer edge of your back foot.

Hold for up to one minute.

To release the pose, press firmly across your back foot. Exhale as you slowly rise to a standing position with your arms stretched at shoulder height. Turn your feet and body so they face the same direction, and then move your feet together. Come back to the top of your mat in the Mountain Pose. Repeat on the opposite side.

Benefits

Increases stamina, strengthens while stretching the legs, knees, and ankles.

Tips

Practice with your back heel against a wall or reach your fingers to a yoga block instead of the arch of your foot to make this exercise easier. Don't forget to keep your chest, legs, and hips aligned.

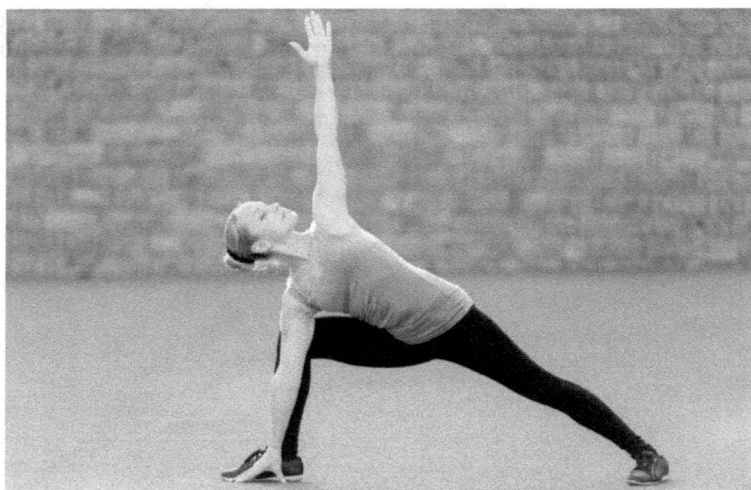

Four-Limbed Staff Pose (Chaturanga Dandasana)

The Four-Limbed Staff Pose is also frequently known as the half-push up. When done correctly, your body resembles a staff or rod, with the spine in one straight line. It is a fundamental component of the Sun Salutations.

How to Do

Bringing your hands shoulder-width apart; supporting your shoulders, elbows, and wrists. Bend your arms straight back, keeping the upper arms hugging into your sides as you lower down toward the floor.

Engage your core and keep your hips raised up creating a line of energy from the crown of your head through your heels. Stop when your forearms and upper arms are at a right angle. So your shoulders are at the same level with your elbows. Hold the pose for ten to thirty seconds, taking four deep breaths. Release with an exhalation.

Benefits

The Four-Limbed Staff Pose tones and strengthens your abs. Builds muscle upper arms, back, and shoulders and wrists.

Tip

For beginners, bring your knees to the floor until you can build enough strength to hold your body up with the arms.

Keep in mind that your neck remains balanced. Your eyes are to the floor. Allowing your body to lower below your elbows can cause elbow strain. If you have wrist conditions, for instance, carpal tunnel syndrome, you should avoid this pose.

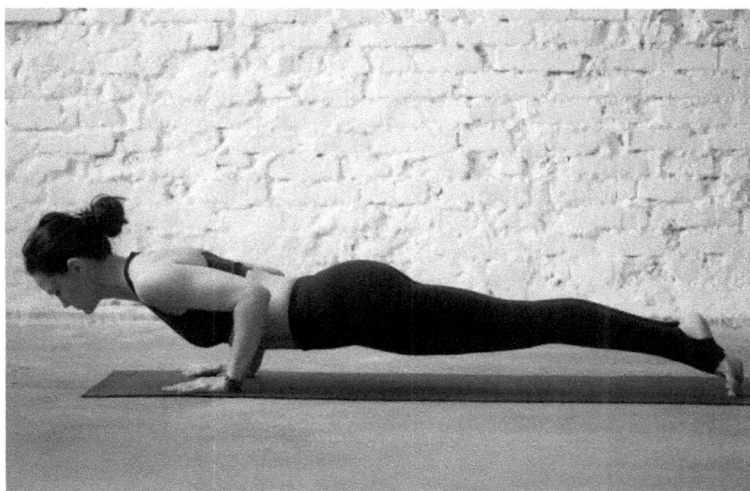

Locust Pose (Salabhasana)

The Locust Pose is a transitional backbend that strengthens and tones the whole back of your body.

How to Do

Lying prone (on your stomach), push your chin against the mat. Keeping your hands in fists with thumbs inside, put your straight arms beneath your thighs. Extend your legs straight behind you, hip-width apart. Make an effort with your back muscles and supporting with your fists from below, use your inner thighs to lift your legs up toward the ceiling, raising both your legs up. Keep this position without holding your breath.

Benefits

The Locust Pose opens your shoulders and neck while it strengthens the back and abdomen. It also eases upper-back aches.

Tips

Roll a blanket and position it at the bottom of your rib cage if you're not gaining much lift in your chest. Practicing like this way will help you strengthen your back muscles.

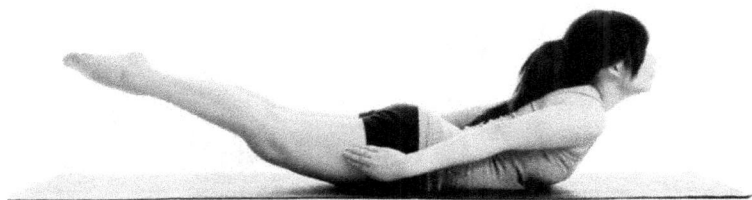

Plank Pose (Kumbhakasana)

As part of the Sun Salutation sequence, the Plank Pose is an arm balancing yoga pose that aids in tightening up your abdominal muscles and strengthening your arms and spine.

How to Do

This pose very similar to as if you were about to undertake a push-up. After completing the Downward Facing Dog, bring your hips forward till your shoulders are over your wrists and your entire body is in one straight line from the top of your head to your heels.

Be sure that your hips don't drop toward the floor or elevated up in the direction of the ceiling. Spreading out your fingers, push them down and balance on your palms. Bend your elbows and remember not to lock them.

Push back through your heels. Shift your shoulders away from your ears. Keeping your neck aligned with your spine, look towards the floor.

Benefits

The Plank Pose tones all the core muscles of the body, including the abdomen, chest, and low back. It strengthens the arms, wrists, and shoulders, and is often used to prepare the body for more challenging arm balances. Plank also strengthens the muscles surrounding the spine which improves posture.

Tips

When practicing the Plank Pose for several minutes, it will help builds endurance and stamina, while toning the nervous system.

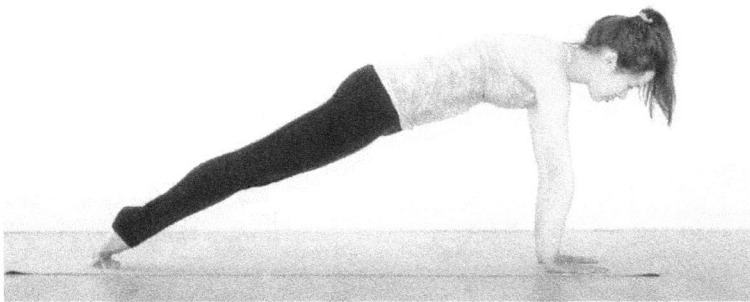

Inverted Triangle Pose (Parivritta Trikonasana)

The Inverted Triangle Pose is one of the more challenging poses for novices as well as advanced practitioners.

How to Do

Begin in the Mountain Pose. Step to the left with your left foot. Pivot your left foot ninety degrees and your right foot about fifteen degrees to the left. Bend your left leg ninety degrees. Extend your arms to your sides, with your palms up. Bend your torso to the left, with your left side facing your left thigh. Reach with your left arm down and right arm up.

Benefits

The Inverted Triangle pose strengthens your leg muscles. It helps sustain a proper balance of your body.

Tips

The Inverted Triangle pose is to some extent easier with a narrower stand. Beginners should likewise, place their hand to the inner foot, either on the floor or on a prop like a block or a chair.

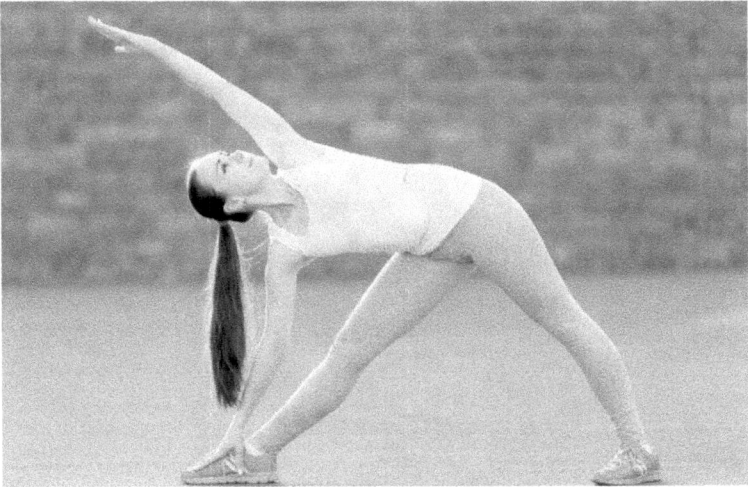

Upward Bow Pose (Urdhva Dhanurasana)

The Upward Bow Pose is considered an advanced yoga pose that stretches and opens your entire body. The Upward Bow Pose can be a difficult pose to attain with the correct alignment.

How to Do

Begin in Corpse Pose. Bending your knees draw your heels toward your hips, positioning them as close as possible to your sitting bones. The bottom of your feet should be hip-width apart and pressed against the floor.

Make ready your body for the pose by raising your hips high off the floor. Drawing your back up into an arch, keep your shoulders steadily planted. Your pose should bear a resemblance to that of the Bridge Pose. Keep this pose for a few breaths, maintaining your pelvis and torso raised and your chin up. Drop your hips back to the floor to get ready for the full bow.

Raise your arms straight up from your sides, starting with the backs of your hands, and bend your elbows as they get nearer to the floor. Place your hands on either side of your head, with your palms down and your fingers pointing toward the shoulders. Your elbows should be pointing up at the ceiling, with your forearms perpendicular to the floor. Keep your elbows pulled inward without crowding around the ears and neck.

Press your feet into the floor and again lift up at the hips as you performed earlier. Hold for a couple of breaths. Push into the hands once more, then breathe in and rise to the top of your head, elevating your shoulders off of the mat. Keep your shoulders squeezed into the back but pulled away from your ears. Maintain this position for a couple of breaths in addition.

At this point, push equally into both your hands and feet, breathe out and raise your head totally off of the ground. Straighten your arms as you lift, maintaining your shoulders and tailbone tightly drawn into the back. Lengthen your legs as your arms straighten out up until you reach the maximum height of your back bend.

Maintain this pose for a few steady breaths, increasing from five to ten-second counts if you're comfortable. To release the pose, lower back down to the top of the head. Put your chin in toward your sternum before lowering your hips and torso to the ground to help you prevent neck injury.

Benefits

The Upward Bow Pose aids in strengthening your legs, the forearms, shoulders, and wrists, helps in toning the buttocks and is an excellent stretch for the biceps and triceps.

This yoga pose is also very helpful in increasing the strength and flexibility of your back, spine, and abdomen.

Tips

Your knees and feet have a tendency to spread as you rise into this pose, which constricts the lower back. In the beginning position, you can loop and secure a strap around your thighs, just above your knees, to hold your thighs at hip width and parallel to each other. To keep your feet from turning out, position a block between them, with the bases of your big toes pressing the ends of the block. You'll find that as you go up, you will press the feet into the block.

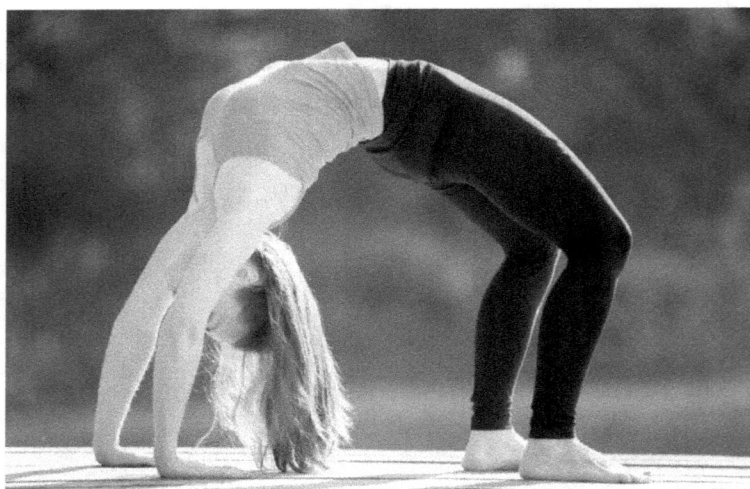

Upward-Facing Dog Pose (Urdhva Mukha Svanasana)

Upward Facing Dog Pose is one of the most generally recognized, as easily as Downward Dog Pose, and recognized yoga pose due to its many benefits and healing purposes. Similar to the Cobra Pose, it is thought of as one of the simplest of the back-bending poses and is regularly carried out during the traditional Sun Salutation sequence.

How to Do

Lie face down on the floor. Extend your legs back, keeping the tops of your feet on the floor. As you bend your elbows, stretch your palms on the floor at the side of your waist, as a result, your forearms are somewhat erect to the floor.

Breathe in and push your inner hands steadily into the floor and slightly back, comparable to trying to force yourself in a forward motion along the floor. Then at the same time, straighten your arms and lift your torso up and your legs a few inches off the floor on an intake breath. Keep the thighs firm and somewhat turned in, the arms steady and turned out to the elbow creases facing forward.

Push your tailbone in the direction of your pubis and lift pubis toward your navel. Contract the hip positions. Stiffen but do not totally harden the buttocks.

Steady your shoulder blades adjacent to the back and puff the side ribs forward. Raise through the upper part of the sternum, however, make an effort not to push the front ribs forward. It will prompt the lower back to tighten. You will at that point look forward or you can angle your head towards the back slightly, remembering to take care not to constrict the back of your neck and the tightening of your throat.

Even though Upward Facing Dog Pose is one of the poses utilized in the classic Sun Salutation Sequence, you can correspondingly practice this pose independently, maintaining the pose fifteen to thirty seconds, inhaling slowly. Release back to the floor or rise into the Downward Facing Dog Pose along with an exhalation.

Benefits

The Upward Facing Dog assists in opening the chest and strengthens the whole body and aligns the spine and invigorates nervous system and the kidneys.

Tips

Performing Upward Facing Dog will elongate and strengthen your whole body. You can utilize it as a backbend by itself, or as a transition for even deeper backbends.

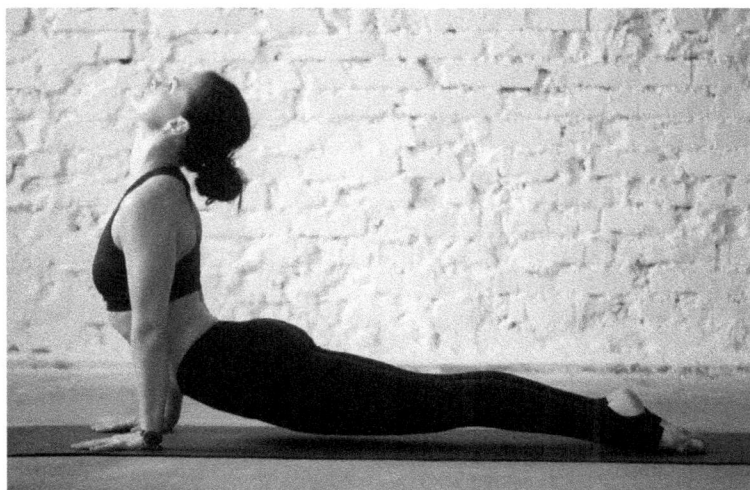

Warrior One Pose (Virabhadrasana)

The Warrior One Pose is the first of a series of three and is a focusing and strengthening pose, aimed to build a link, grounding you with the Earth's energy.

How to Do

Move your right foot toward the back of your mat to come into Warrior I. Bring your right heel to the floor and turn your right toes out to about a forty-five-degree angle. Bend your left knee over the left ankle. You might need to correct the length of your stance from the front to back. You can also broaden your stance from side to side for a greater stability. Maintain the position of your hips that same as it was in Mountain pose, with the hips pointing forward.

While breathing in, bring your arms up over your head. Your arm position may vary in relation to the flexibility in your shoulders. The typical position is with the palms touching above, but you may decide on keeping your palms apart at shoulder distance or you can bend at your elbows and open your arms resembling a saguaro cactus. A slight backbend will open the heart and the gaze move toward the fingertips.

Benefits

The Warrior One Pose helps strengthen and tone your arms, legs and lower back. It also helps increase stamina and improves the balance in your body.

Tips

Warrior One Pose has been shown with the heel of your front foot aligned with the arch of your back foot as if you were on a balance beam. This division enables the hips to square more.

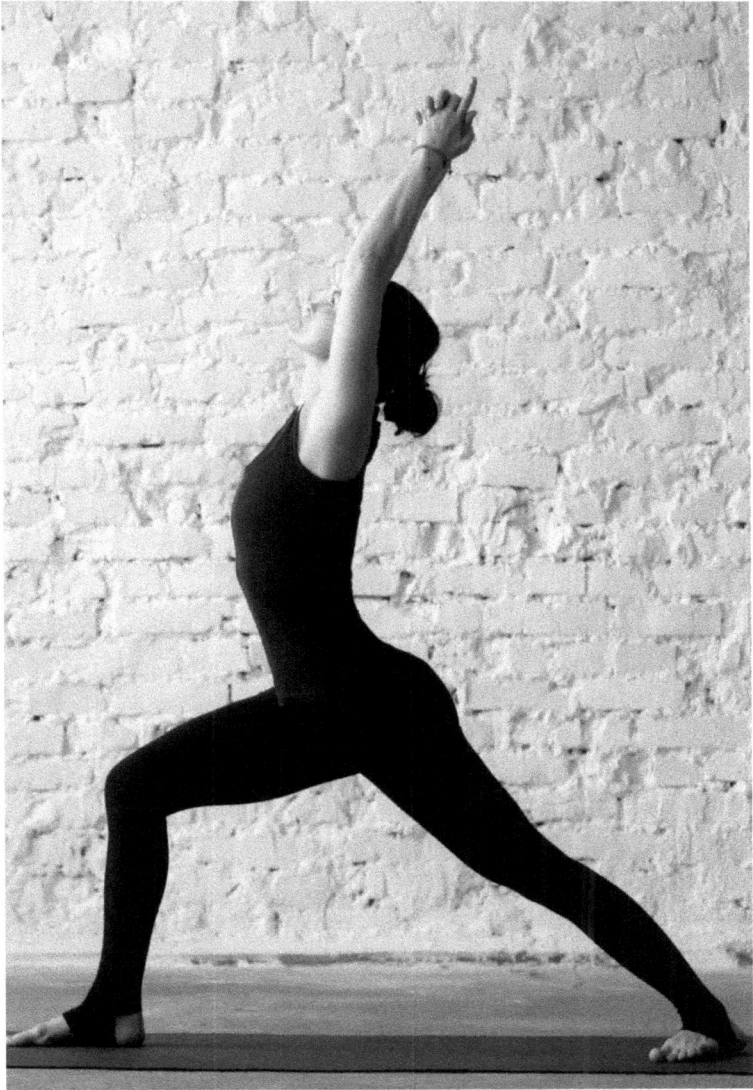

Warrior Two Pose (Virabhadrasana II)

The Warrior Two Pose is the second of a sequence of three yoga poses that improve strength and stamina.

How to Do

From the Downward Facing Dog, step your left foot to the inside your left hand. Bend your left knee over your ankle so your thigh is parallel to the floor. Swivel on the ball of your right foot to bring your right heel to your mat. Your right foot should be at a 90-degree angle with the sole planted.

Your front heel is lined up with your back arch. Rise to stand. Open your hips to the right side of your mat. Your torso will face right. Extend your left arm toward the front of the mat and your right arm toward the back of the mat with your palms facing down. Keep both arms parallel to the floor. Release your shoulders away from your ears. Reach out through the fingertips of both hands.

Turn your head to face the front of your mat. Your gaze is forward over the left hand. Both thighs are rotating outward.

Engage your triceps to support your arms, your quadriceps to support your legs, and your belly to support your torso.

After several breaths, windmill your hands down to either side of your left foot and step back to Downward Dog. Stay here for a few breaths or go through a transition before repeating the pose with the right foot forward.

Benefits

Tones the abdomen, strengthen your legs and arms and opens your chest and shoulders.

Tips

When you bend the right knee to a right angle, bend it with a meaningful exhalation, and point the inside the right knee in the direction of the little-toe side of the right foot.

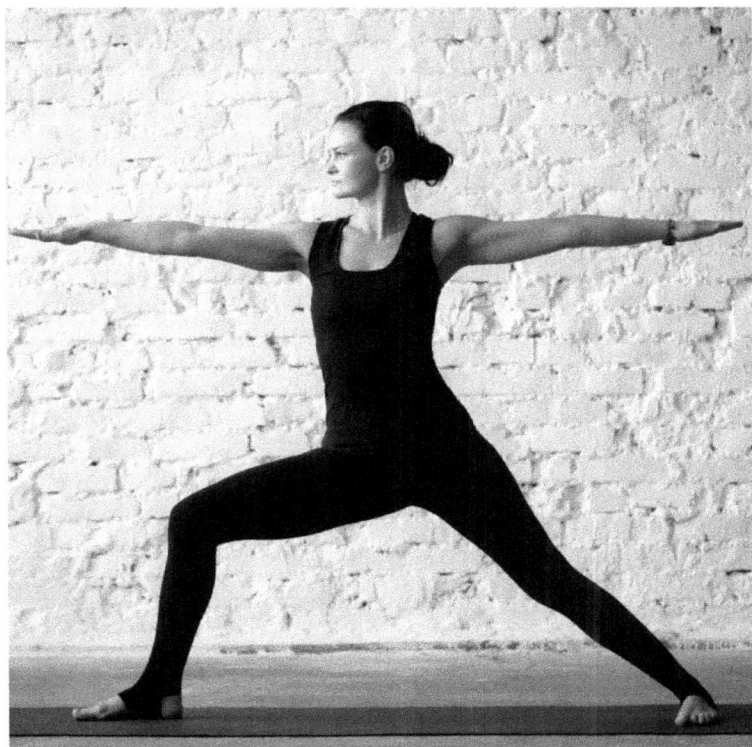

Warrior Three Pose (Virabhadrasana III)

The Warrior Three Pose is an intermediate balancing pose in yoga. This energetic standing posture builds stability throughout your whole body by incorporating all of the muscles through your core, arms, and legs.

How to Do

Begin in the Mountain Pose. With an exhale, move your right foot back about two feet, as you maintain your body weight forward on your left foot. Keep your left toes looking forward. Feel your left toes spread and find an even basis through the sole of your left foot. Put your hands on your hips to bring into line your hips and shoulders perpendicular to the front of your mat. Tighten your inner core muscles by pulling in the navel and waist.

Maintain a feeling you are holding the lower organs with a round band of muscle, then breathe in and raise your right foot as your incline your torso forward experiencing a hinging movement at your hips. Direct your stare straight down as you bend forward from your hips attaining a new focus.

As your torso and right leg go into a corresponding position with the floor, lengthen both legs without bracing into the bottom knee. The right hip may rise higher than the left. Keeping your right hip level with the left hip, experience a shift in a correct postural alignment. Imagine more length advancing into the right leg and spine. Maintain the digging into the left foot and tightening into the core muscles.

To intensify the influence of the balance, free your hands from your hips and elongate your arms straight out to the sides expanding your chest or forward in line with your head and neck. If you extend your arms forward, then turn your palms to face each other so your shoulder blades can draw down away from your ears. Breathe and stay here for five to ten breaths.

To release this pose, inhale as you lift your chest and place your right foot back into Mountain Pose. Exhale as you lower your arms, and draw a few breaths as you pause and then repeat on the right side for the same time.

Benefits

The Warrior III pose strengthens your legs, improves balance and your core strength.

Tips

You can either stand in front of the wall, bringing your arms outstretched in front of you with your hands on the wall or rotate and bring the raised back foot onto the wall. Both will give you the stability you require to level your hips. You can also hold on a chair as a substitute for using the wall.

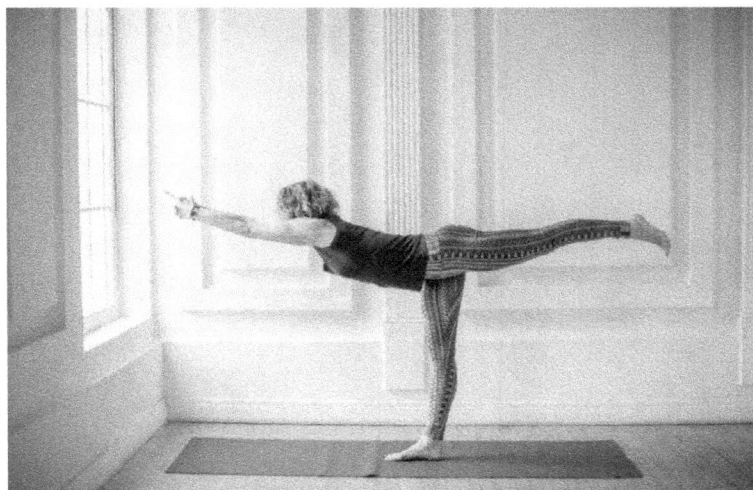

Seated Forward Fold Pose
(Paschimottanasana)

The Seated Forward Fold is a calming yoga pose that aids to relieve stress. This pose is frequently performed later in a series, when the body is warm.

How to Do

From the Staff Pose, inhale the arms up over the head and lift and lengthen up through the fingers and crown of the head. Exhale and bend at the hips, slowly drop your torso towards your legs. Reach the hands to the toes, feet or ankles.

To deepen the stretch, use the arms to gently pull the head and torso closer to the legs. Press out through the heels and gently draw the toes towards you. Breathe and hold for five to ten breaths. To release from this pose slowly roll up the spine back into Staff pose. Inhale the arms back over your head as you lift the torso back into the Staff pose.

Benefits

The Seated Forward Fold delivers a deep stretch for the whole back side of your body from the heels to the neck. The Forward Fold soothes your nervous system and emotions.

Tips

By no means should force yourself into a forward bend, particularly when sitting on the floor. Extend forward, when you feel the area between your pubis and navel shortening, you should stop, lift up a little, and lengthen again. Frequently, because of the tightness in the backs of your legs, a beginner's forward bend doesn't go very far forward and may possibly look more like sitting up straight.

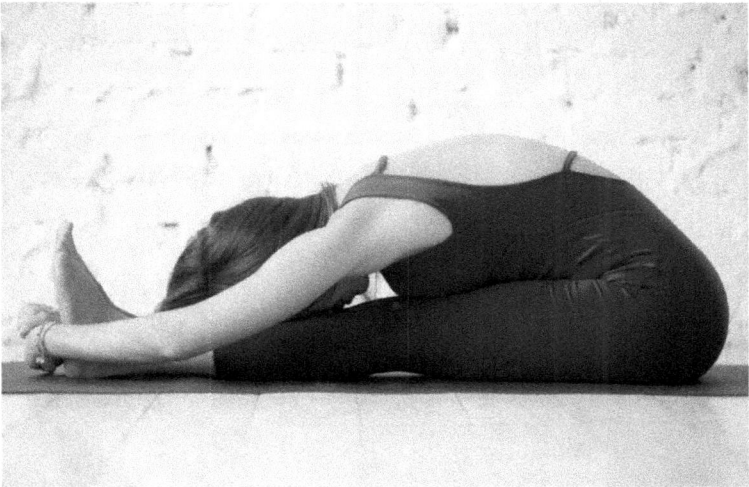

Bow Pose (Dhanurasana)

The Bow Pose is an invigorating pose in which the practitioner lays on their belly, grabs their feet, and lifts the legs into the shape of a bow.

How to Do

Lie on your stomach (prone) with your arms by your side and palms facing upwards. Roll your shoulders on your back so that the tops of your arm bones rise off the floor and your shoulder blades move towards each other. Bend both your knees so that your feet move towards your buttocks.

Clasp your ankles with your hands. You can arch your feet to make a handle. You do not want hold your foot itself. Breathe out and tighten through your abdominal area with the principle of lengthening your lower back and bring support to your spine. Breathe in and lengthen out through the top of your head, while, at the same time, maintaining your knees hip width apart, press your feet back into your hands, forming a natural lift.

With each breath, press your heels back and up, gradually increasing the back bend, keeping the spine elongated. Maintain the effective contraction of the abdominal muscles to counter any pressure that may go into the lower spine.

Hold for 5 breaths or more. Exhale and slowly release the feet. Lie quietly for a few moments. You can repeat if desired.

Benefits

The Bow Pose strengthens your abdominal muscles, adds greater flexibility to the back. It tones the leg and arm muscles, opens up the chest, neck, and shoulders and it is also a useful stress and fatigue buster.

Tips

Place a firm blanket or pillow underneath your hip bones for extra padding, if you need it. To prevent ankle, knee, and other leg injuries, hold onto your ankles, not the tops of your feet.

If it isn't possible for you to clasp your ankles completely, use a strap around the fronts of your ankles and fasten the free ends of the strap, as you maintain your arms fully stretched out.

Remember to keep breathing throughout the pose. Do not hold your breath.

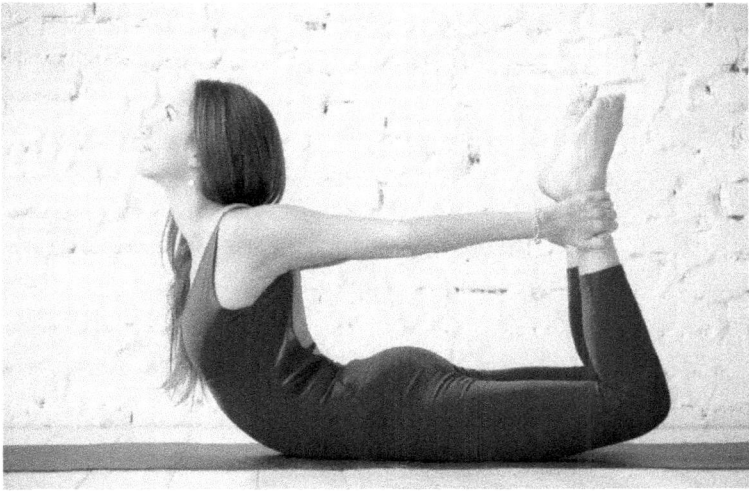

Standing Forward Fold Pose (Uttanasana)

Standing Forward Fold Pose is an important component of the Sun Salutations. This pose is used to train the body for deeper forward bends.

How to Do

Begin by Standing with your feet together. Bend your knees somewhat and bend your torso, not the lower back, over your legs, shift from your hips. Put your hands on the floor in front of you or next to your feet.

Breathe in and expand your chest to elongate your spine. Keep your focus fixed forward.

Breathe out and press both legs straight. Raise your kneecaps and twist your upper and inner thighs back. Without hyperextending, maintain your legs straight.

Extend your torso down without rounding your back, on an exhalation. Stay long through your neck, lengthening the top of your head toward the ground. Pull your shoulders down your back.

Benefits

The Standing Forward Fold pose extends your spinal column and stretches the back muscles as well as the backs of your legs.

Tip

Bend your knees to increase the stretch in the backs of your legs. Take care not to straighten the knees by locking them back; as an alternative, allow them to straighten as the two ends of each leg move farther spaced out.

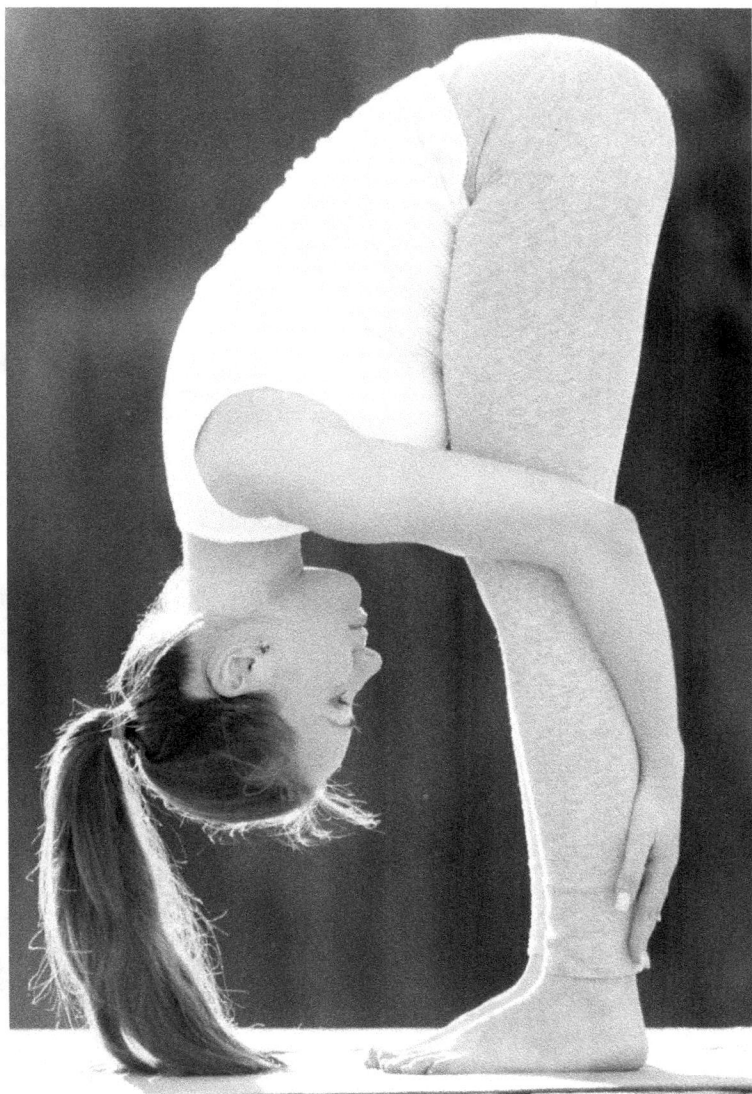

Butterfly Pose (Baddha Konasana)

The Butterfly Pose is a seated pose that strengthens and opens your hips and groin while decreasing abdominal pain.

How to Do

Sit with your knees near to your chest. Relax your knees out to each side and slightly press the bottoms of your feet together. Hold on to your ankles or feet.

Benefits

The Butterfly Pose is a good stretch for your inner thighs, groins, and knees. It helps improve the flexibility in your groin and hip area. When standing and walking for long hours, it removes fatigue.

Can give assistance from menstrual discomfort and menopause symptoms and smooth delivery if it's practiced on a regular basis until late pregnancy. Also helps in intestine and bowel movement.

Tips

You may find it difficult to lower your knees toward the floor. If your knees are incredibly high and your back is rounded, be sure to sit on a high support, even as high as a foot off the floor.

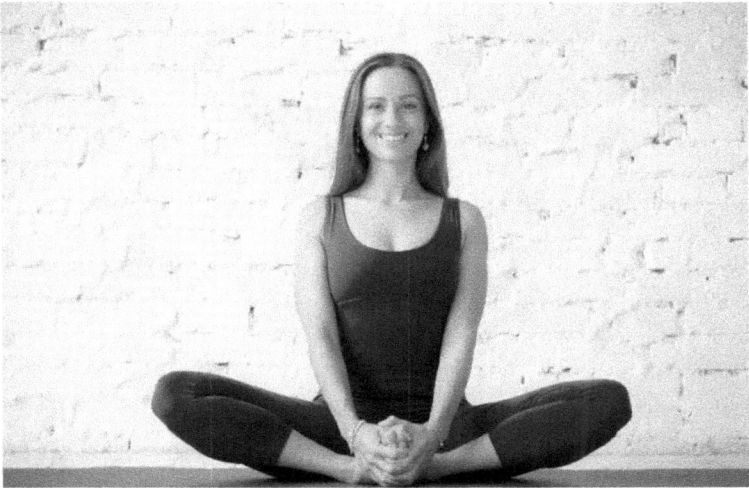

Bridge Pose (Setu Bandha Sarvangasana)

The Bridge Pose is a beginning backbend that helps to open your chest and stretch your thighs.

How to Do

To begin, lie supine (on your back). Fold your knees and keep your feet hip distance apart on the floor, ten to twelve inches from your pelvis, with your knees and ankles in a straight line. With your arms beside your body, place your palms faced down.

Breathe in, while slowly lifting your lower back, middle back and upper back off the floor. Gently roll in your shoulders. Touch your chest to your chin without bringing the chin down. Support your weight with your shoulders, arms, and feet. Feel your buttocks firm up in this pose. Both your thighs should be parallel to each other and to the floor.

You could interlock your fingers and push your hands on the floor to lift your torso a bit more up if you want or you could support your back with your palms. Keep breathing easily.

Hold this pose for a minute or two and then exhale as you gently release the pose.

Benefits

The Bridge Pose strengthens your back, opens the chest, and improves your spinal mobility.

Tips

After you roll your shoulders under, be sure not to pull them away from your ears. This often overstrains your neck. Raise the tops of your shoulders toward your ears and push your inner shoulder blades away from your spine.

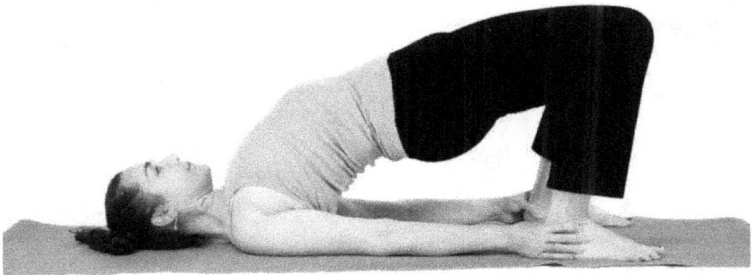

Child's Pose (Balasana)

The Child's Pose is a popular beginner's yoga posture. It is generally utilized as a resting position in among more difficult poses throughout a yoga practice.

How to Do

Come to all fours (Table Pose) exhale and lower your hips to your heels and forehead to the floor. Kneeling on the floor, bring your big toes together and sit on your heels, then separate your knees about as far as your hips.

Your arms can be above your head with your palms on the floor. Your palms can be flat or fisted with them stacked under your forehead, or your arms can be at the sides of your body with your palms up.

The Child's Pose is a resting pose. Remain in this position anywhere from thirty seconds to a few minutes. Beginners can also use this pose to get a feel of a deep forward bend. To come up, first stretch your front torso, followed by an inhalation lift from your tailbone as it pushes down and into your pelvis.

Benefits

The Child's Pose aids to stretch your hips, thighs, and ankles at the same time it reduces stress and fatigue. It gradually relaxes the muscles on the front of your body while softly and reflexively elongates the muscles of the back of your torso.

As it centers, calm, and soothes your brain, the Child's Pose is said to be a beneficial posture for alleviating stress. When done with your head and torso braced, it can as well help relieve back and neck pain.

The Child's Pose soothes the body, mind, and spirit while stimulating your third eye. Gently stretching the lower back, the Child's Pose massages and tones your abdominal organs, and encourages digestion and elimination.

Tips

Before you relax completely, press your palms into the ground with your arms straight and elbows lifted. Push your hips firmly back toward your heels. Breathe deeply into your whole back, for an extra release in your back. Make use of this pose to rest in the middle of more challenging poses.

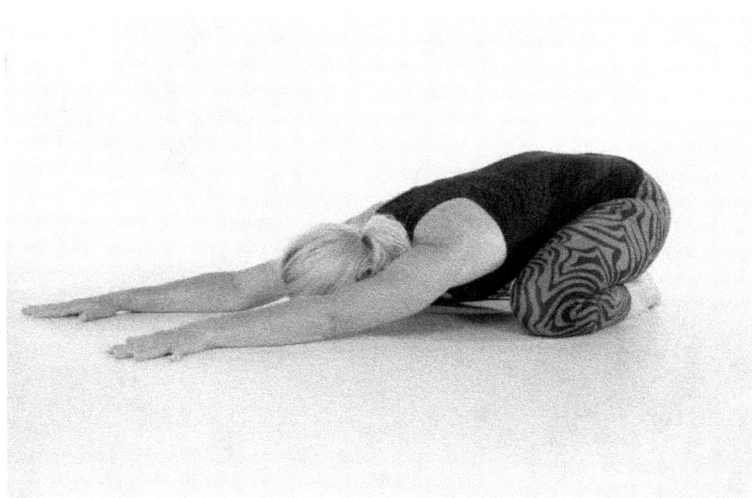

Constructing a Yoga Sequence

Here are a few points to keep in mind how to construct a yoga sequence. You are not at a studio, paying to be there. You do not have to exercise for over an hour. Begin with 5-10 minutes. Notice how you feel by the end of this time. If you feel as if you can do more, go ahead. If no, end your routine there.

Start with 5-10 minutes. By the conclusion of that time, notice how you feel. Do you desire to resume? If yes, continue for an extra five minutes and then check in with yourself once more. If not, close your workout.

The same as any physical journey, a yoga sequence has three clear parts.

Your opening or warm-up sequence

You don't want to jump into the main event tight and cold. This is where you move through and loosening up your major muscle groups as well as body parts

Your main sequence

Once you've warmed up, it's time for your main sequence. This component of your sequence is influenced by the goal of your routine. If it's an asymmetrical pose, keep in mind to do both sides and devote about the same time on each side.

The closing or cool down sequence

Now you've completed the principal portion of your yoga practice, it's time to cool down.

About The Author

Monique Joiner Siedlak is a writer, witch, and warrior on a mission to awaken people to their greatest potential through the power of storytelling infused with mysticism, modern paganism, and new age spirituality. At the young age of 12, she began rigorously studying the fascinating philosophy of Wicca. By the time she was 20, she was self-initiated into the craft, and hasn't looked back ever since. To this day, she has authored over 35 books pertaining to the magick and mysteries of life. Her most recent publication is book one of an Urban Paranormal series entitled "Jaeger Chronicles."

Originally from Long Island, New York, Monique is now a proud inhabitant of Northeast Florida; however, she considers herself to be a citizen of Mother Earth. When she doesn't have a book or pen in hand, she loves exploring new places and learning new things. And being the nature lover that she is, she considers herself to be an avid animal advocate.

To find out more about Monique Joiner Siedlak artistically, spiritually, and personally, feel free to visit her **official website**.

Other Books by Monique Joiner Siedlak

Mojo's Wiccan Series

Wiccan Basics

Candle Magick

Wiccan Spells

Love Spells

Abundance Spells

Hoodoo

Herb Magick

Seven African Powers: The Orishas

Moon Magick

Cooking for the Orishas

Creating Your Own Spells

Body Mind and Soul Series

Creative Visualization

Astral Projection for Beginners

Meditation for Beginners

Reiki for Beginners

Thorne Witch Series

The Phoenix

Beautiful You Series

Creating Your Own Body Butter

Creating Your Own Body Scrub

Creating Your Own Body Spray

Mojo's Self-Improvement Series

Manifesting With the Law of Attraction

Stress Management

Jaeger Chronicles

Glen Cove

Connect With Me!

I really appreciate you reading my book! Please leave a review and let me know your thoughts. Here are the social media locations you can find me at:

Like my **Facebook Page**: www.facebook.com/mojosiedlak

Follow me on **Twitter**: www.twitter.com/mojosiedlak

Follow me on **Instagram**: www.instagram.com/mojosiedlak

Follow me on **Bookbub**: http://bit.ly/2KEMkqt

Sign up to my **Email List** at www.mojosiedlak.com and receive a free book!

If you enjoyed this book or found it useful I'd be very grateful if you'd post a short review on at your retailer. Your support really does make a difference and I read all the reviews personally so I can get your feedback and make this as well as the next book even better.

www.ingramcontent.com/pod-product-compliance
Lightning Source LLC
Chambersburg PA
CBHW071340290326
41933CB00040B/1824